Skicinuwi 'Pisunol

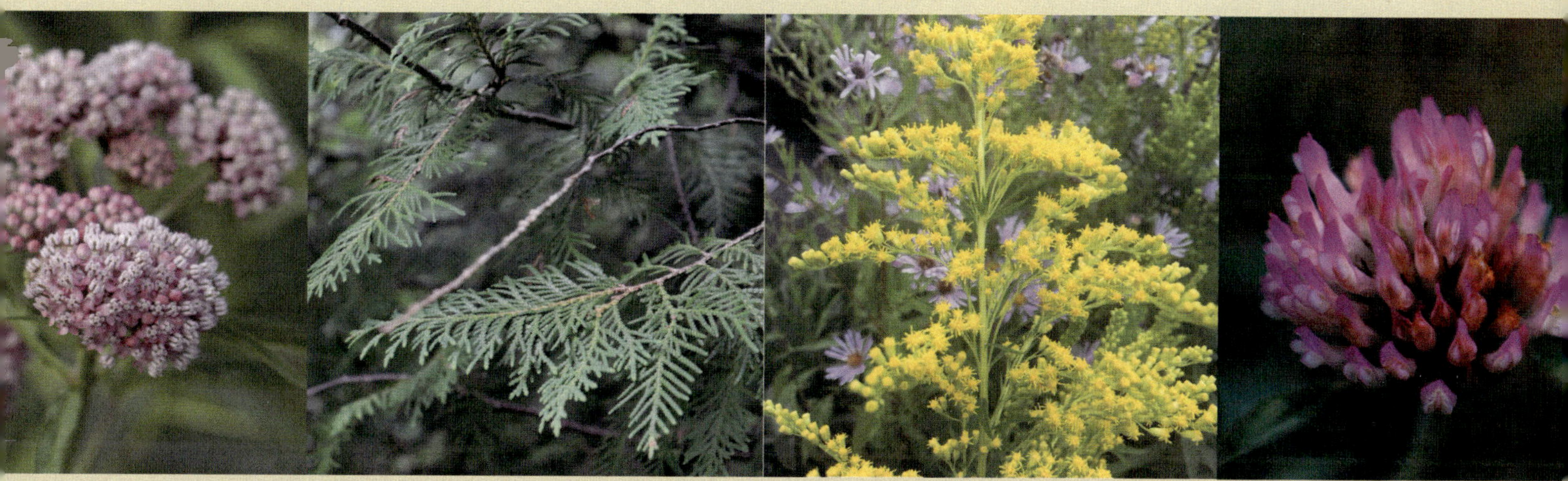

Neqotkuk N'tetli Mikwi Tahasoltipen
&
Wolastoq Ed

Language Translator: Neqotkuk Elder

KAKSKUS

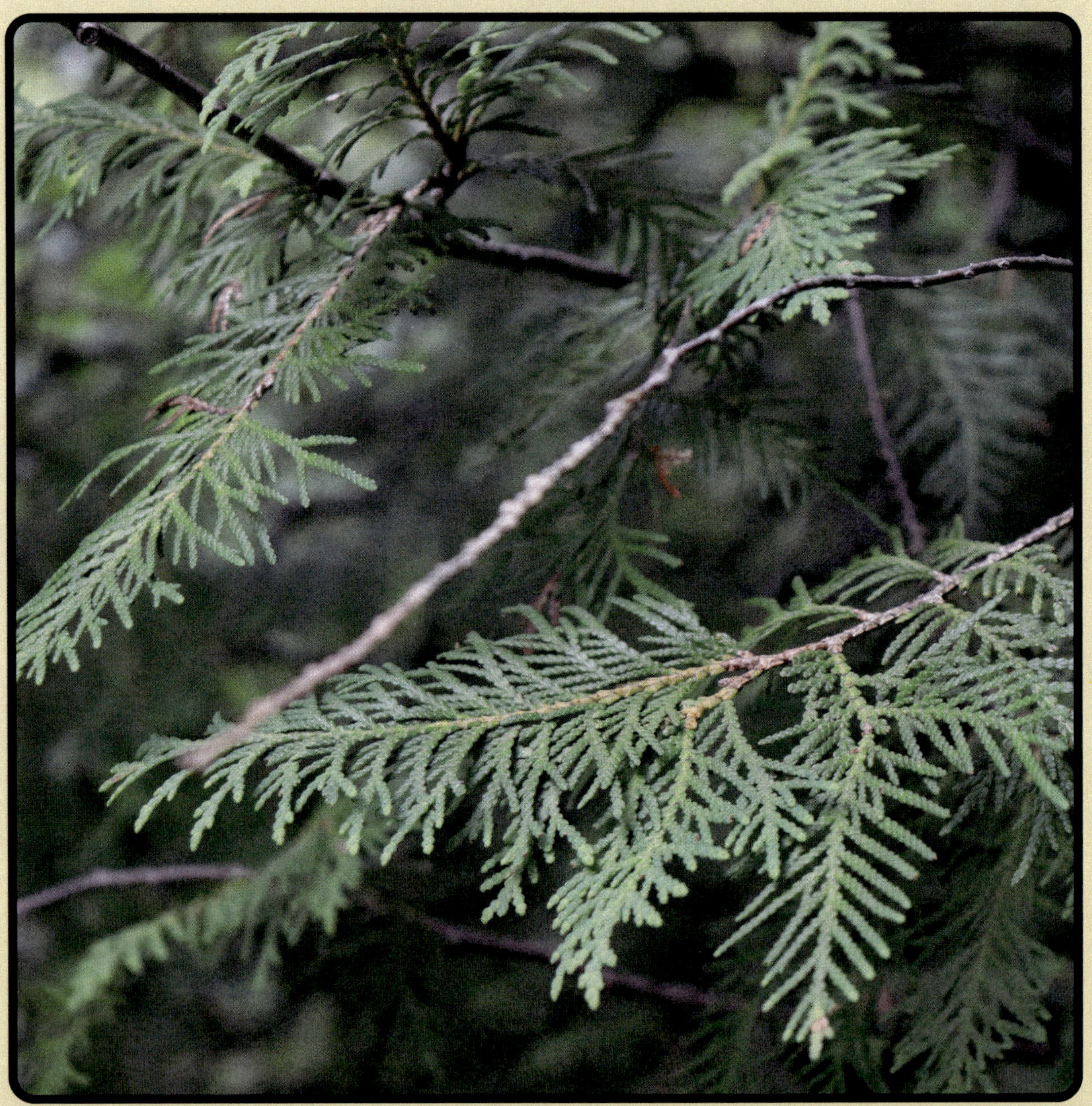

Cedar

Blooms: Siqonomeqi-kisuhs (May)

Harvest time: When leaves are a vibrant green and new growth is evident

Medicinal uses: Traditionally, as a tea, it would help reduce fevers, rheumatic symptoms and relieve symptoms of chest colds and the flu. The green leaves are high in vitamin C and used to create a salve that is nourishing to the skin. Kakskus (cedar) is considered purifying and is very important to the Wolastoqiyik and Mi'kmaw, who often use it for ceremonies and sweat lodges.

CIKONESISOK

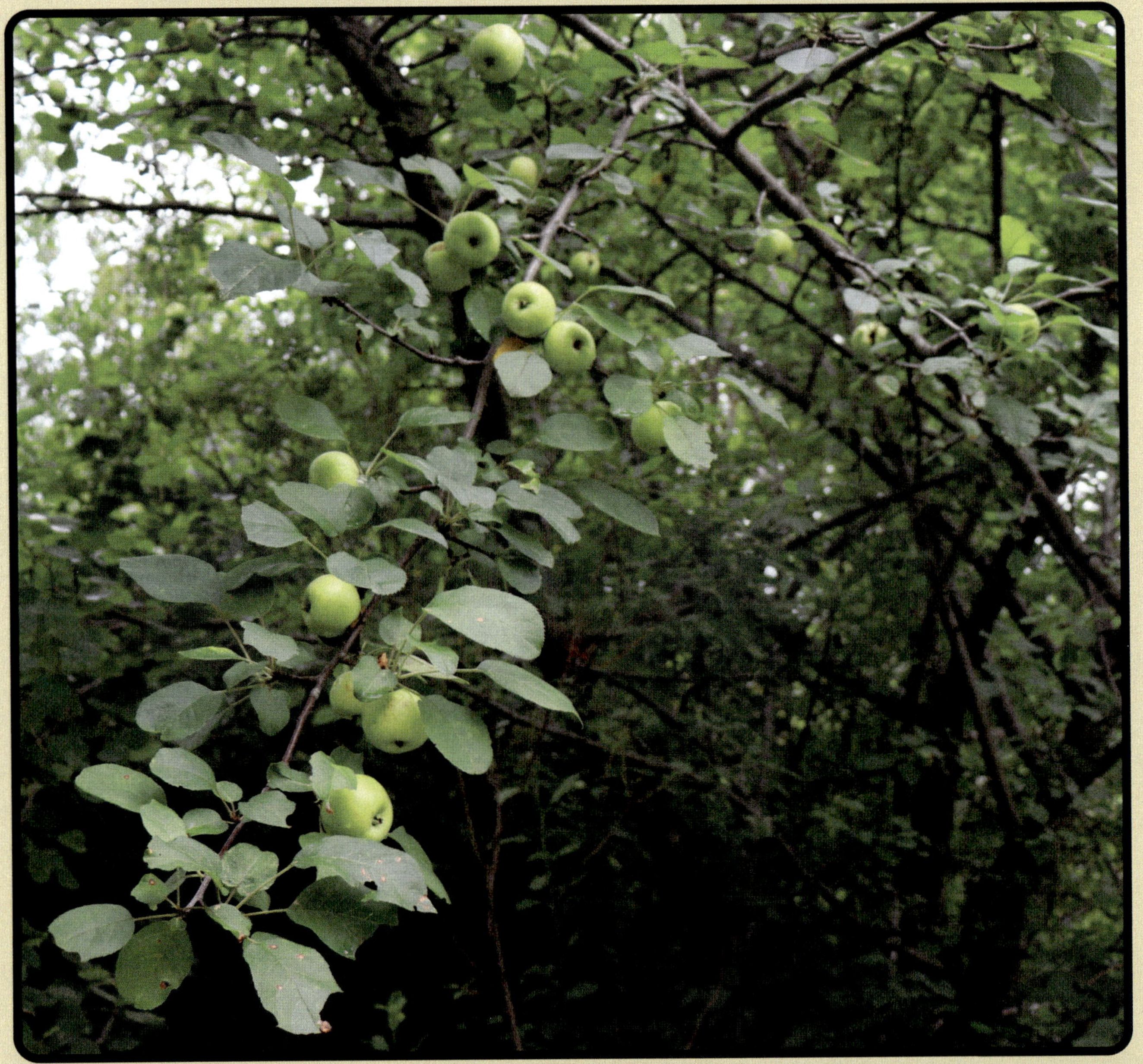

Crab Apple Tree

Blooms: Spring - Summer (Siqoniw - Niponiw)

Harvest time: Puniw (Winter)

Medicinal uses: Stimulates the digestive system and protects against constipation. The fruit pulp can be used to heal inflammations or small flesh wounds.

POMUHSE IMIYAMKEWEY

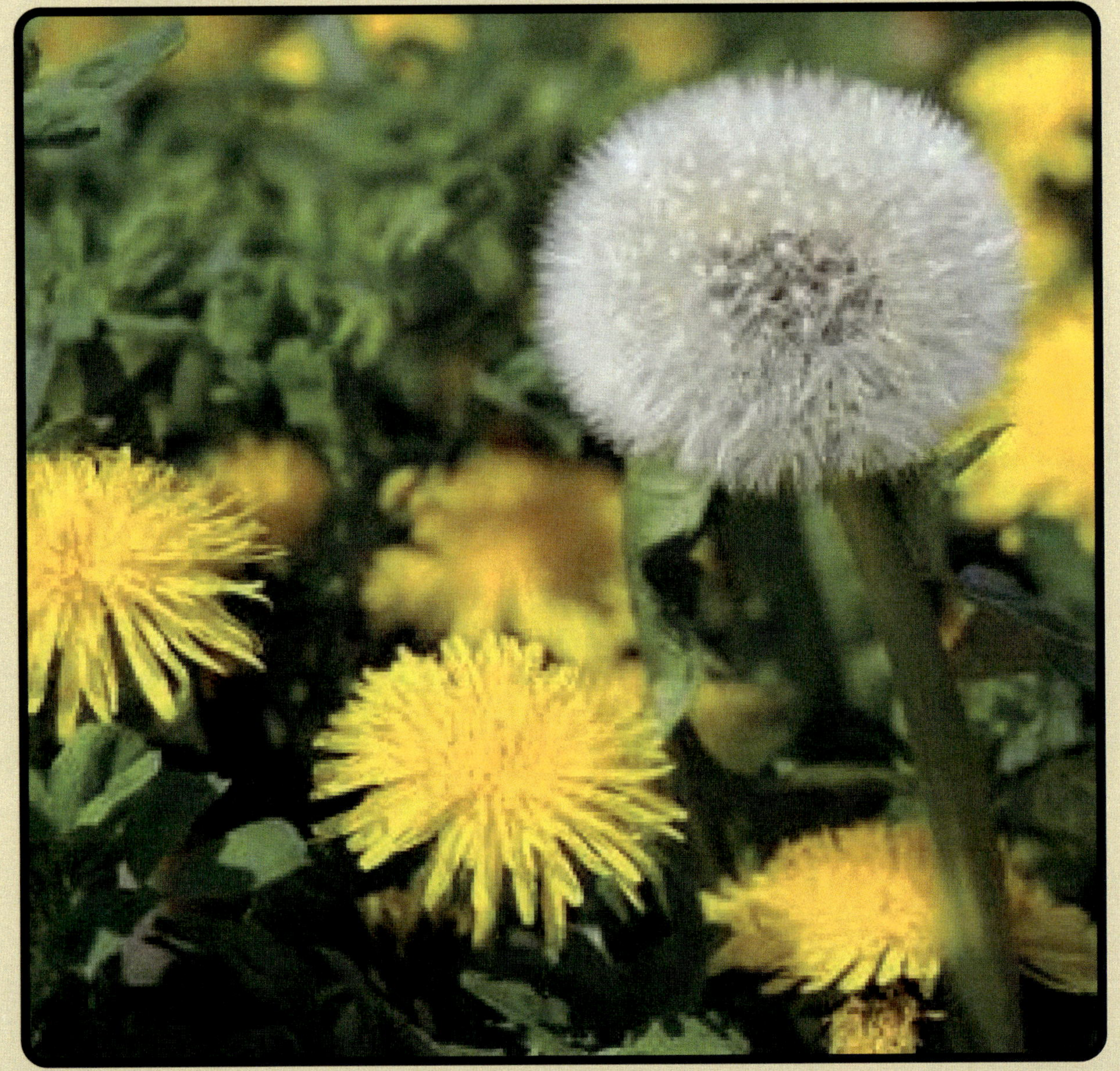

Dandelion

Blooms: Siqonomeqi-kisuhs - Amilkewi-kisuhs (May to October)

Harvest time: When leaves are still small and tender in early spring, preferably before the flower comes out

Medicinal uses: When boiled it can be used to treat kidney disease, swelling, skin problems, heartburn and upset stomach. It could be used as a digestive aid and to help strengthen the immune system. It is also used as a diuretic to increase the amount of urine and eliminate fluid in your body to help problems such as liver issues and high blood pressure.

UNIYAS

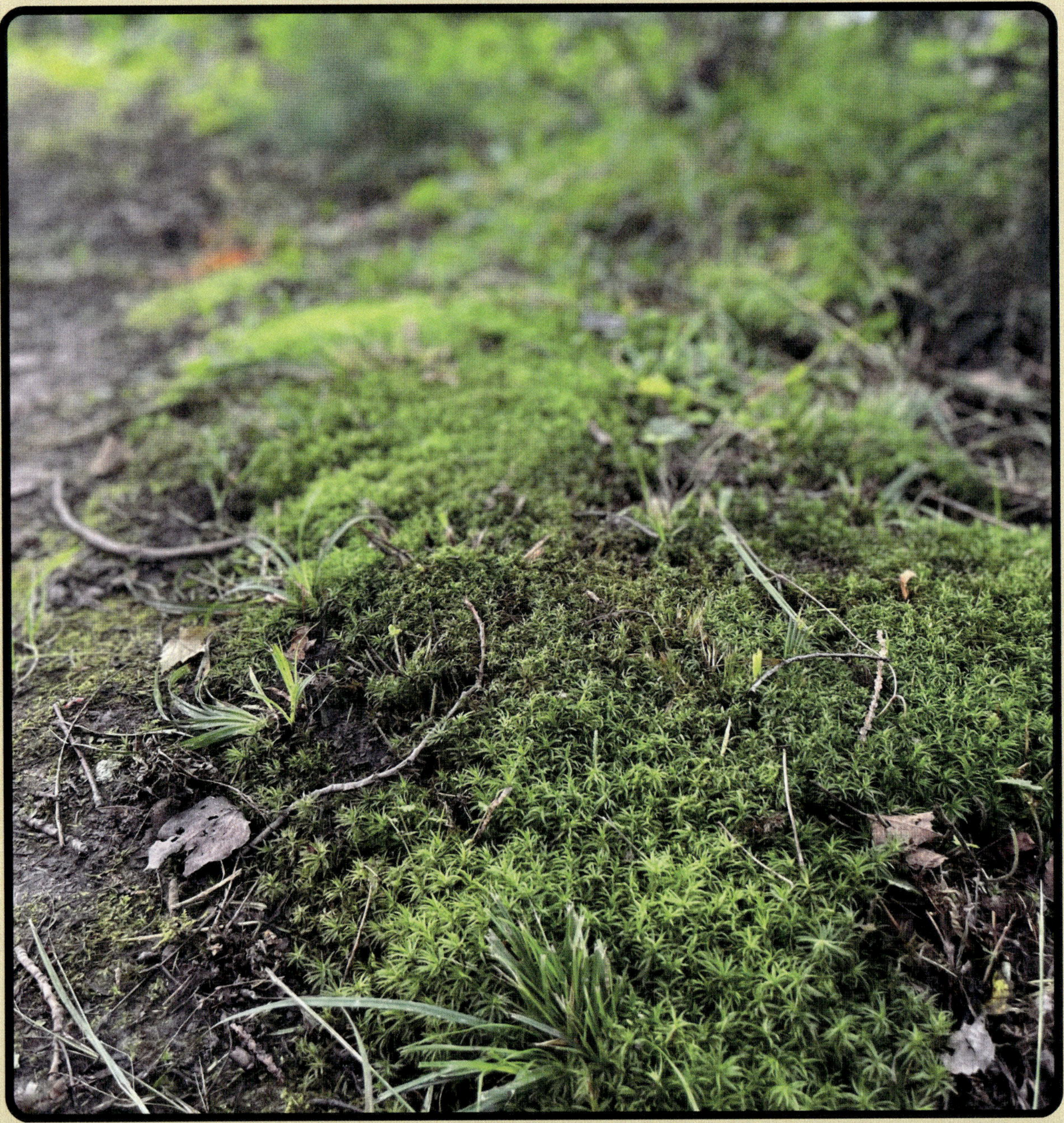

Moss

Blooms: Niponiw - Toqakiw
(Summer - Fall)

Harvest time: Ideally when it's moist, and a patch without too much grass or other plants

Medicinal uses: Most commonly used as a cure for coughs or as a diuretic, it depends on how the moss is processed and which moss is used.

WISAWKESKIL

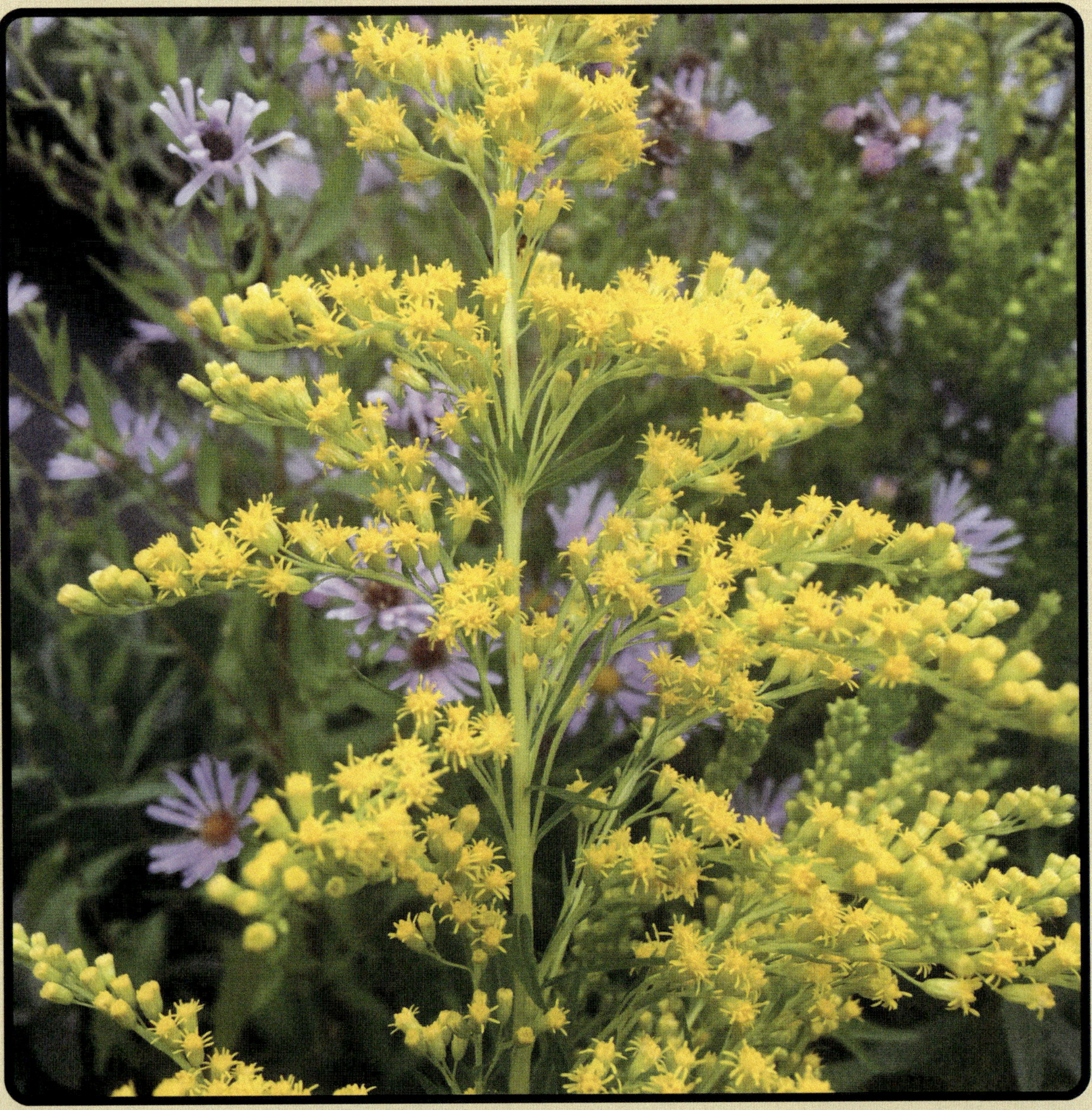

Canada Golden Rod

Blooms: Apsqewi-kisuhs - Amilkewi-kisuhs (July - October)

Harvest time: In the toqakiw (fall) after the first heavy frost it is best to harvest

Medicinal uses: To treat tuberculosis, diabetes, enlargement of the liver, gout, hemorrhoids, internal bleeding, asthma, and arthritis. It can be used as a mouth rinse to treat inflammation of the mouth and throat. It can also be used to make tea or dietary supplements from the roots, the leaves and seeds can be eaten but must be cooked or boiled first.

SOLANIMUS

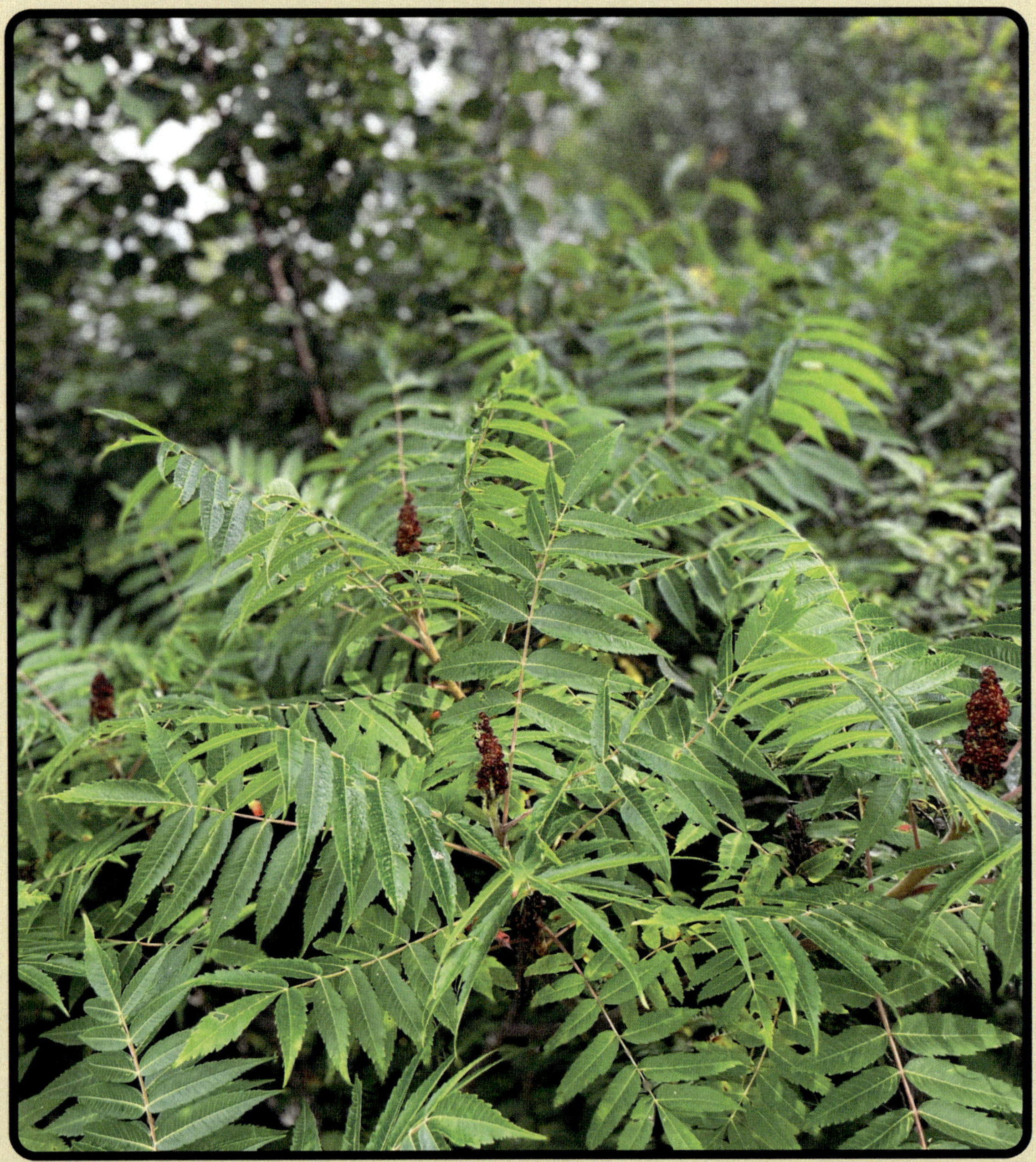

Sumac

Blooms: Siqonomeqi-kisuhs - Apsqewi-kisuhs (May - July)

Harvest time: Amoniyat-kisuhs - Amilkewi-kisuhs (August - October)

Medicinal uses: To treat colds, sore throats, fever, infections, diarrhea, dysentery and scurvy. Sumac has also been used to treat asthma and cold sores, and lower blood sugar.

PULOSAHSIS

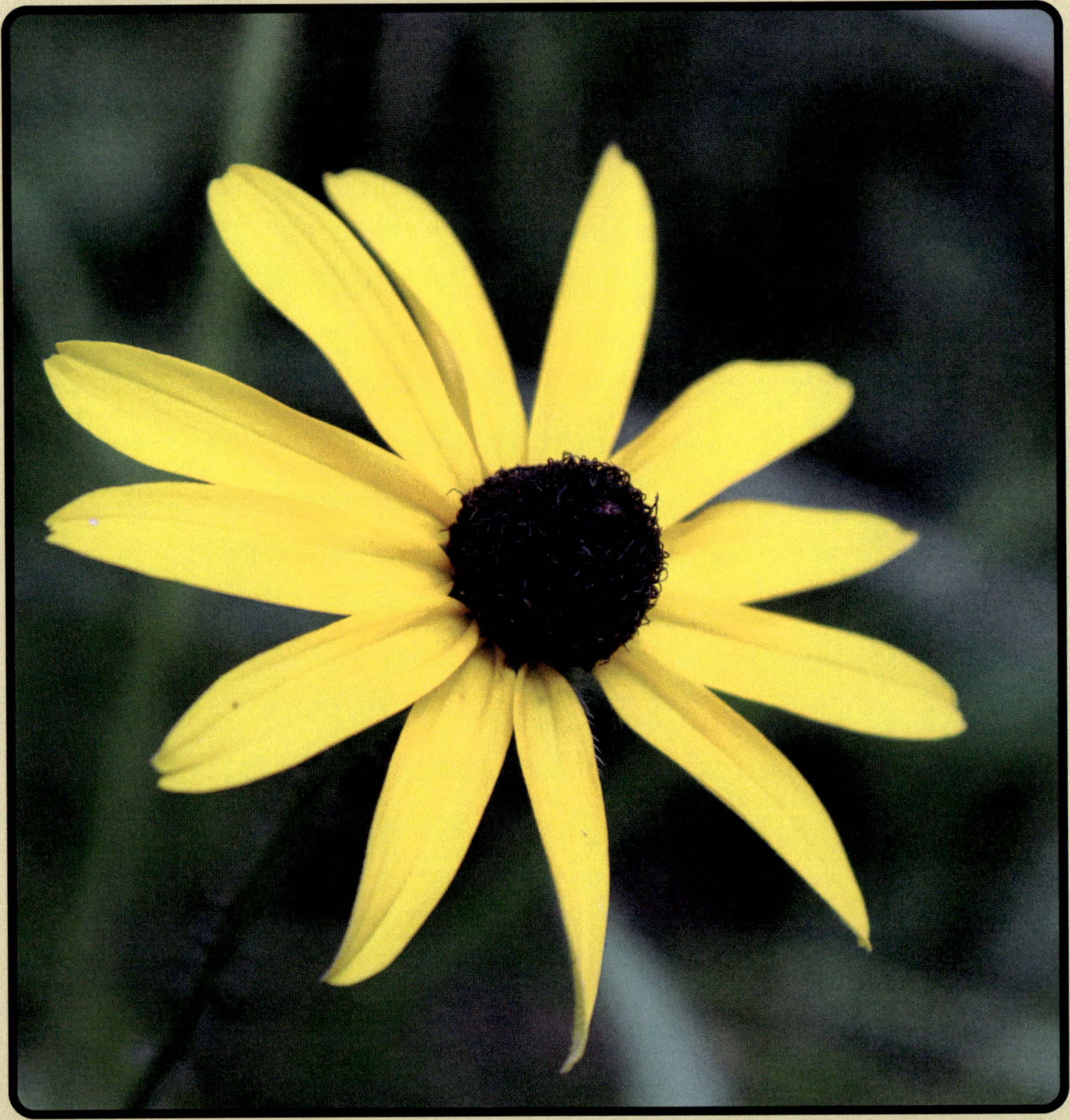

Black-eyed Susan

Blooms: Niponi-kisuhs - Toqaquwi-kisuhs (June - September)

Harvest time: Siqoniw (Spring)

Medicinal uses: To treat the common cold and flu, as well as strengthen the immune system, help treat high blood pressure, diuresis, and ulcers. It can also be used to treat earaches, snake bites, and to get rid of parasitic worms.

MASQEMUS

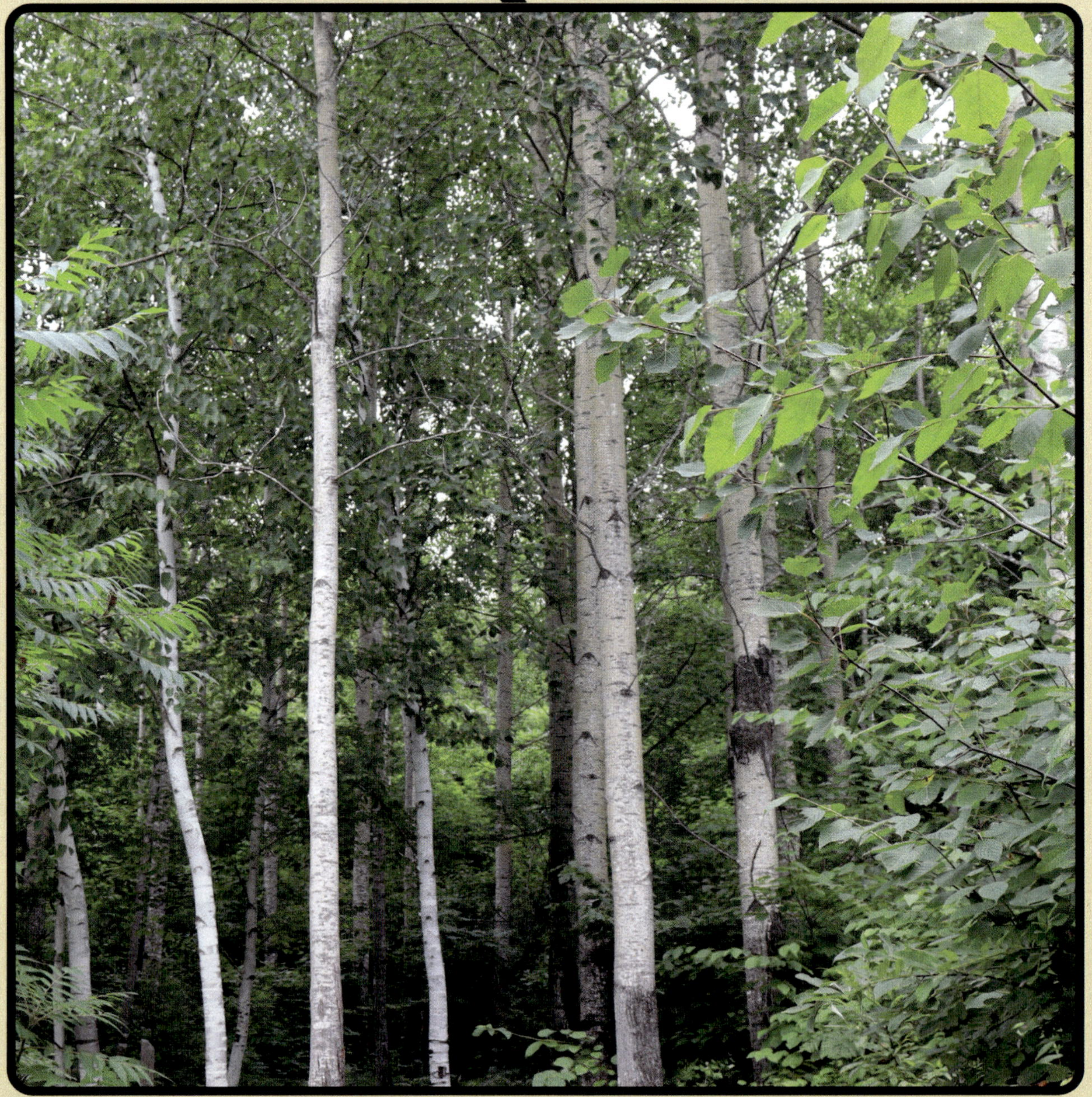

Paper Birch Tree

Blooms: Siqoniw (Spring)

Harvest time: Siqoniw when sap is running through the tree, and must be cautious not to damage the inner bark.

Medicinal uses: To treat rheumatism, arthritis, gout, calcium spurs, heart and kidney edema, chronic cystitis, colds, coughs, and high cholesterol. Making a tea out of the bark, twigs, and dried leaves can be used as an anti-inflammatory.

NESPIHQAMKUK

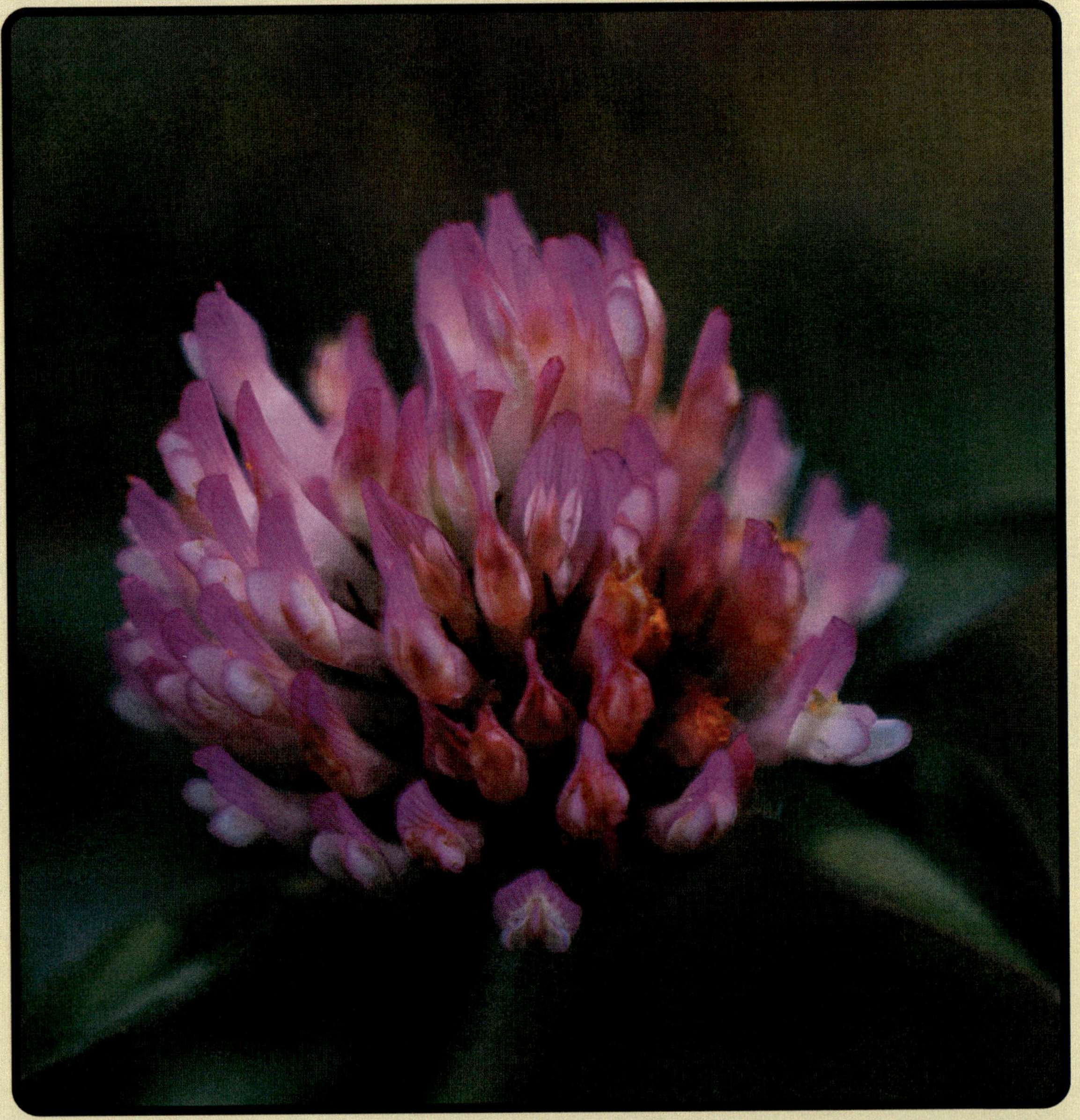

Red Clover

Blooms: Siqoniw - Niponiw (Spring - Summer)

Harvest time: When the seeds begin to turn brown and the flower heads dry out. After they have dried, you can harvest them by cutting off the entire stem above the soil line.

Medicinal uses: Treats respiratory symptoms (asthma, whooping cough, and bronchitis), skin disorders (eczema and psoriasis), inflammatory disorders (arthritis), and women's health issues (menopausal and menstrual symptoms).

PASKTEHSON

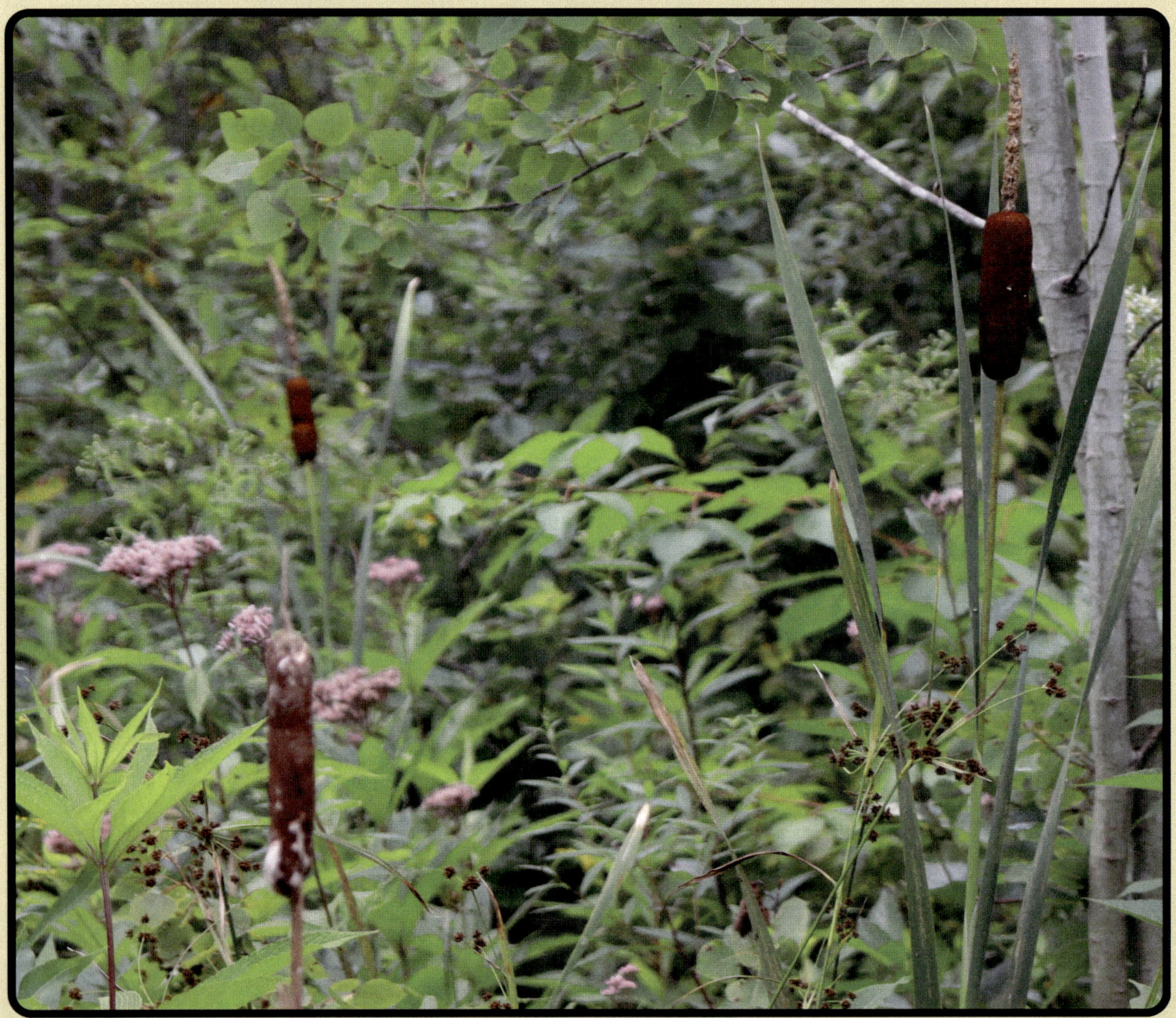

Cattails

Blooms: Siqoniw (Spring)

Harvest time: Toqakiw (Fall)

Medicinal Uses: Treat wounds, burns, stings, and bruises. The ash of the burned pasktehson leaves can be used as an antiseptic or styptic for wounds. A small drop of a honey-like excretion, often found near the base of the plant, can be used as an antiseptic for small wounds and toothaches.

KAWIS

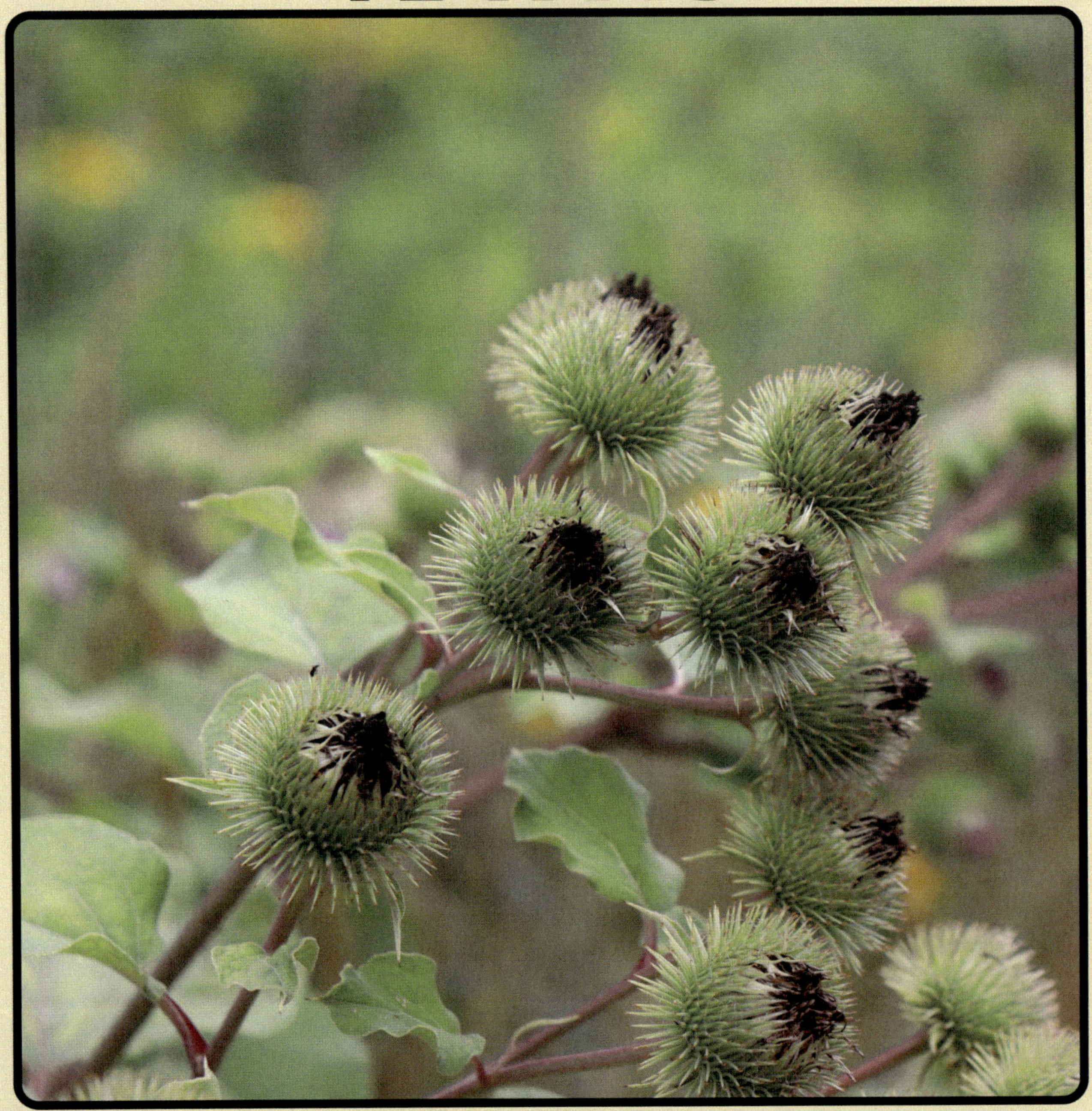

Burdock

Blooms: Niponiw - Toqakiw (Summer - Fall)

Harvest time: After the first hard frost of the year

Medicinal uses: Increases urine flow, kills germs, reduces fever, and purifies blood. It is also used to treat colds, cancer, anorexia nervosa, gastrointestinal (GI) complaints, joint pain (rheumatism), gout, bladder infections, complications of syphillis, and skin conditions including acne and psoriasis.

MOLAQSIYAK

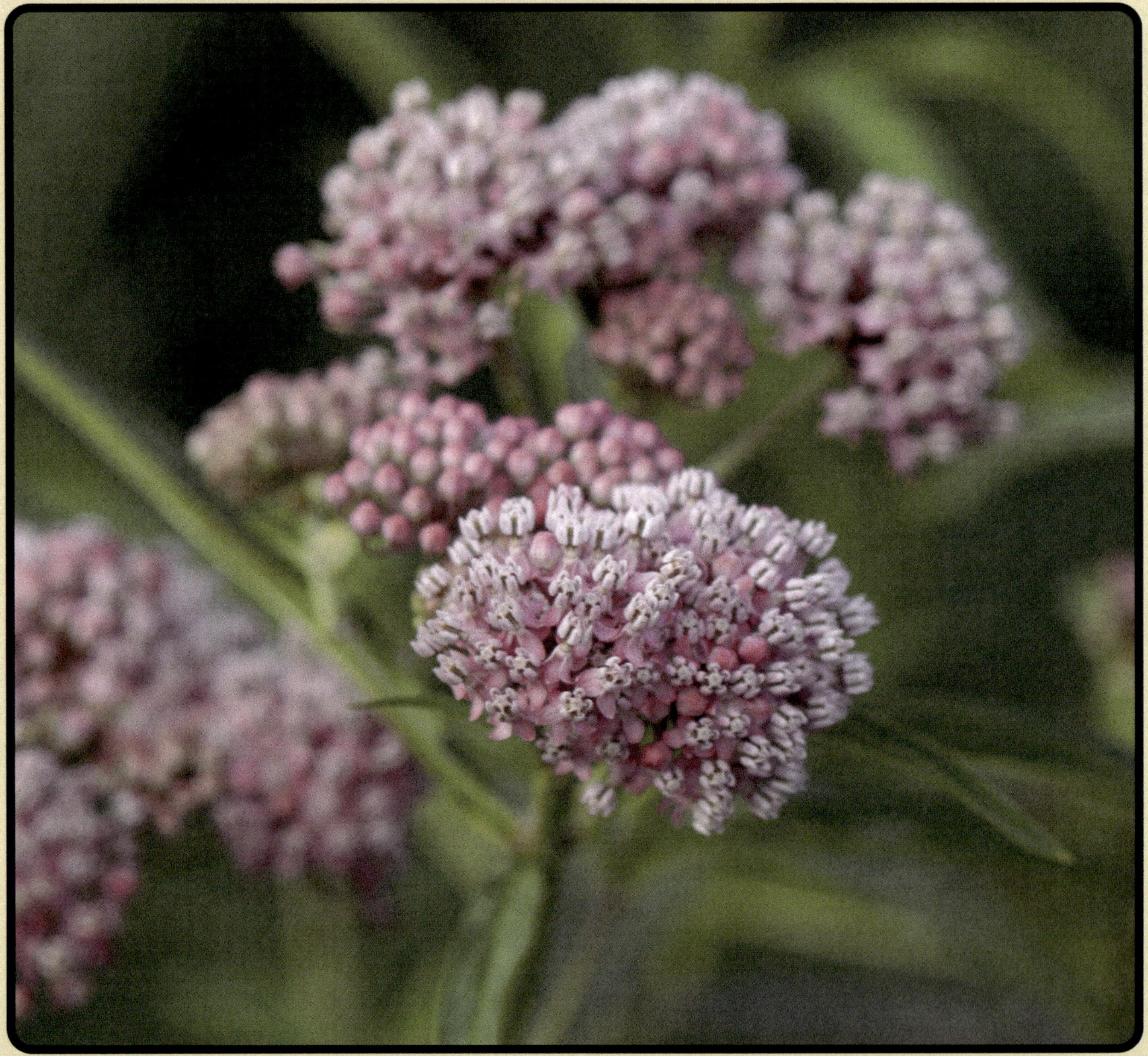

Swamp Milkweed

Blooms: Siqoniw - Niponiw (Spring - Summer)

Harvest time: Toqakiw (Fall)

Medicinal uses: When made into a tea, it can be used to destroy parasitic worms, relieving flatulence, to help kidneys produce more urine, promote appetite, assist digestion and act as a laxative. It can also be used in the treatment of asthma, syphillis, rheumatism, and as a heart tonic.

MEHQAQSOSKIL

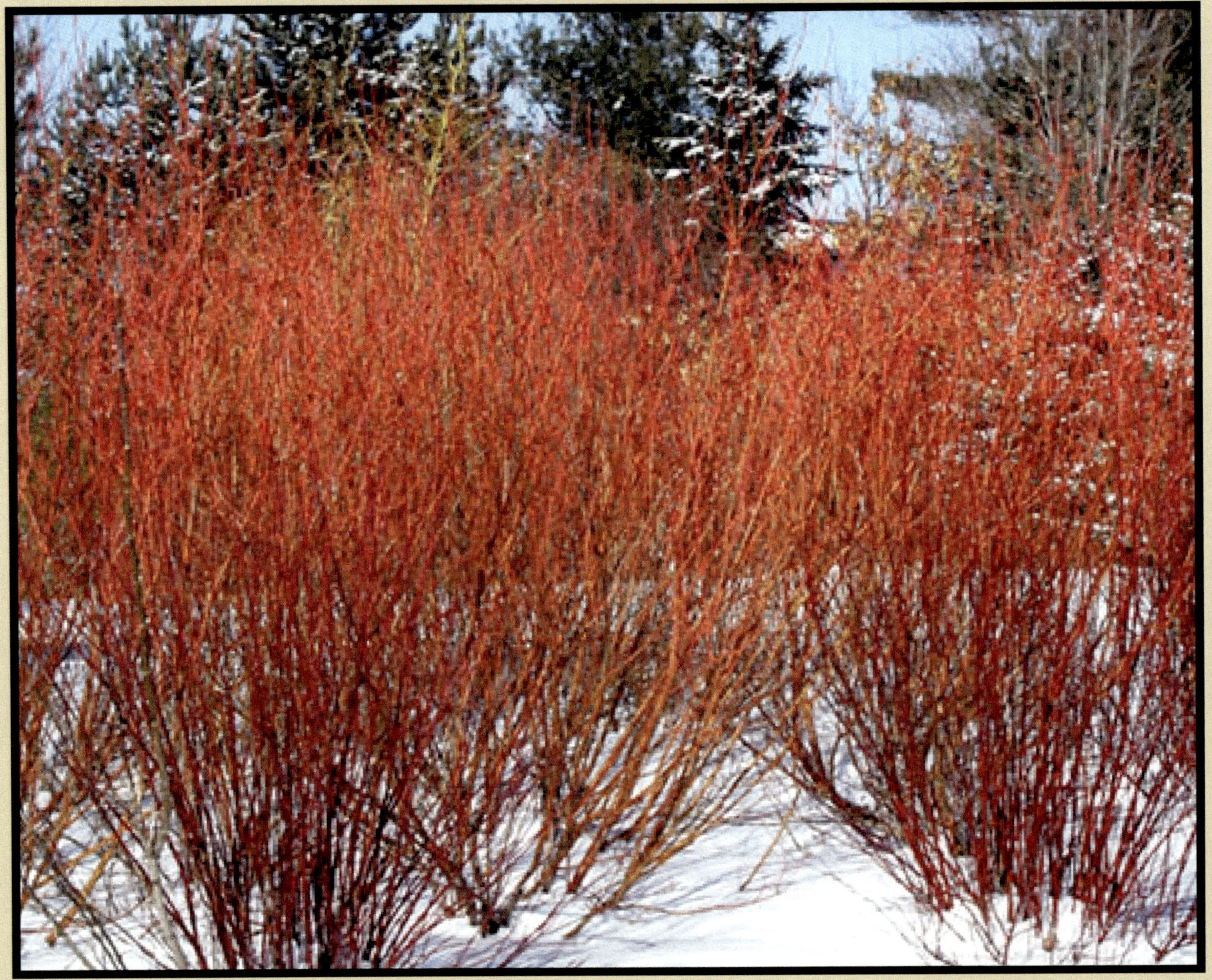

Red Osierdogwood

Blooms: Siqonomeqi-kisuhs - Niponi-kisuhs (May - June)

Harvest time: In the Siqoniw (spring) before the leaves come out, and in the Toqakiw (fall) after the leaves have shed

Medicinal uses: A tea made from the bark has been used internally for coughs, colds, fevers, sinus congestion, liver problems, and postpartum bleeding. Externally the bark tea has been used as a wash for rashes, ulcers, and dandruff.

SIPISEY KALT LO

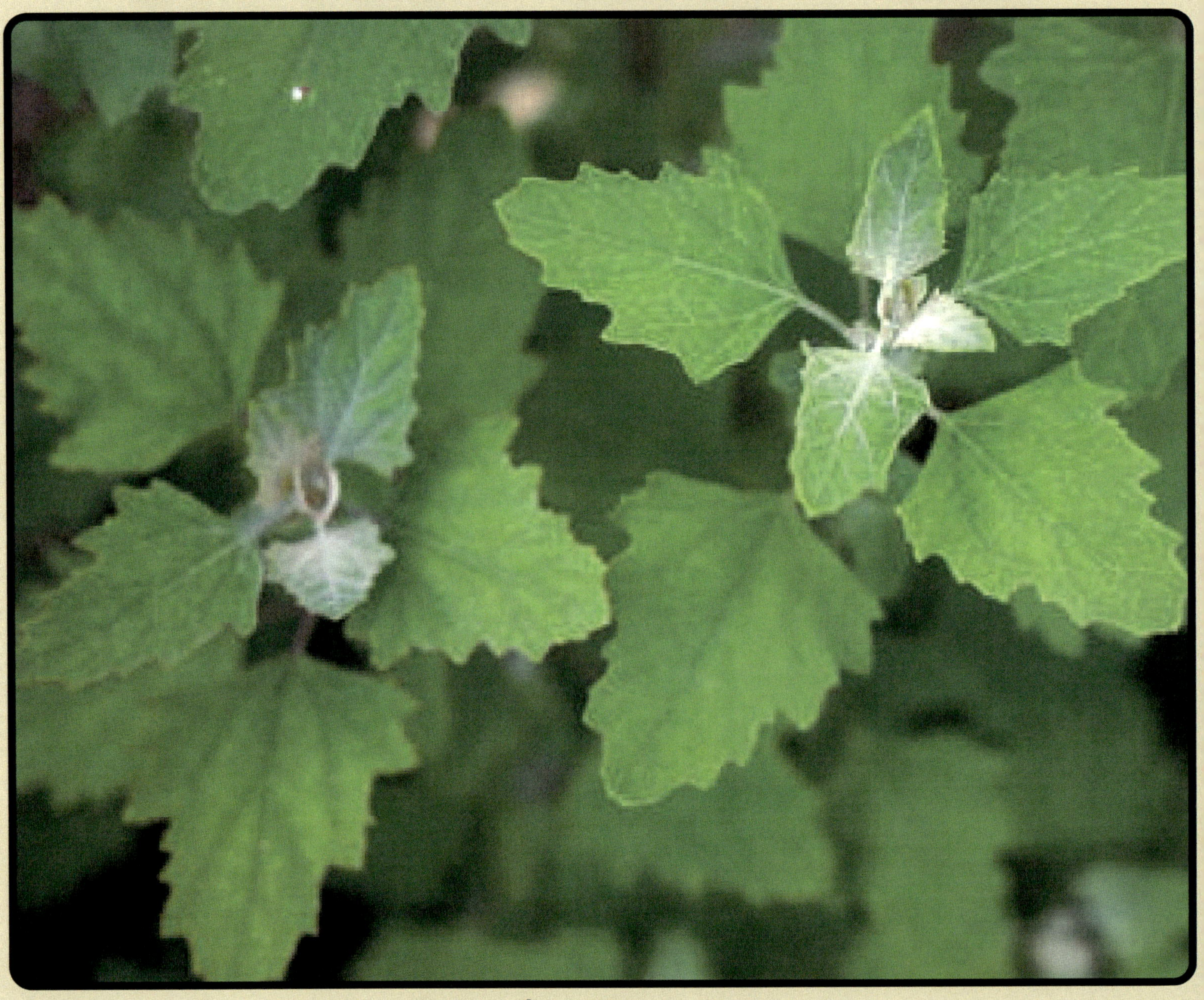

Lambs Quarter

Blooms: Niponiw - Toqakiw (Summer - Fall)

Harvest time: All year round in the morning ideally but best time is when the plant is young and tender

Medicinal uses: Lambs quarter is an important source of food that can be considered to be a key staple, while at the same time it is also an extremely valuable medicine. When the leaves are chewed into a green paste and applied to the body, it makes a great poultice to treat insect bites, minor scrapes, injuries, inflammation, and sunburn. Also, it contains high levels of Vitamin C which can help cure scurvy.

MACIPOSIT MITIYEY

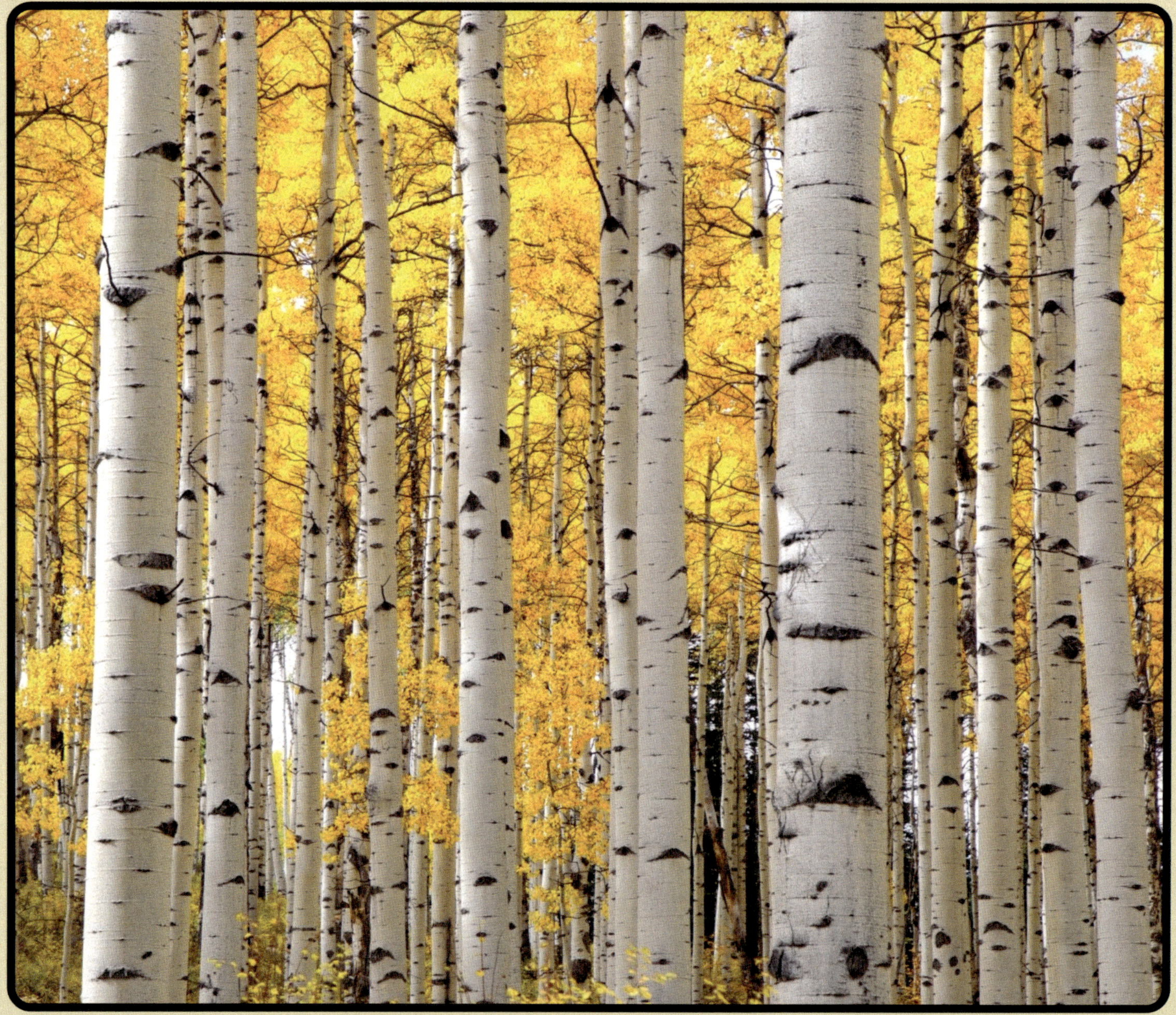

Trembling Aspen

Blooms: These flowers are produced in early (spring) before the leaves grow on trees.

Harvest time: All year round but best time is when the first capsule begins to split open and white puppus (fluff) begins to break out.

Medicinal use: The bark could be boiled into cough medicine (syrup). Boil the roots for debilities. Boil the buds with fat for a salve for a cold. The root was eaten by women to prevent premature childbirth and heart medicine.

KINAPITAT MITIYEY

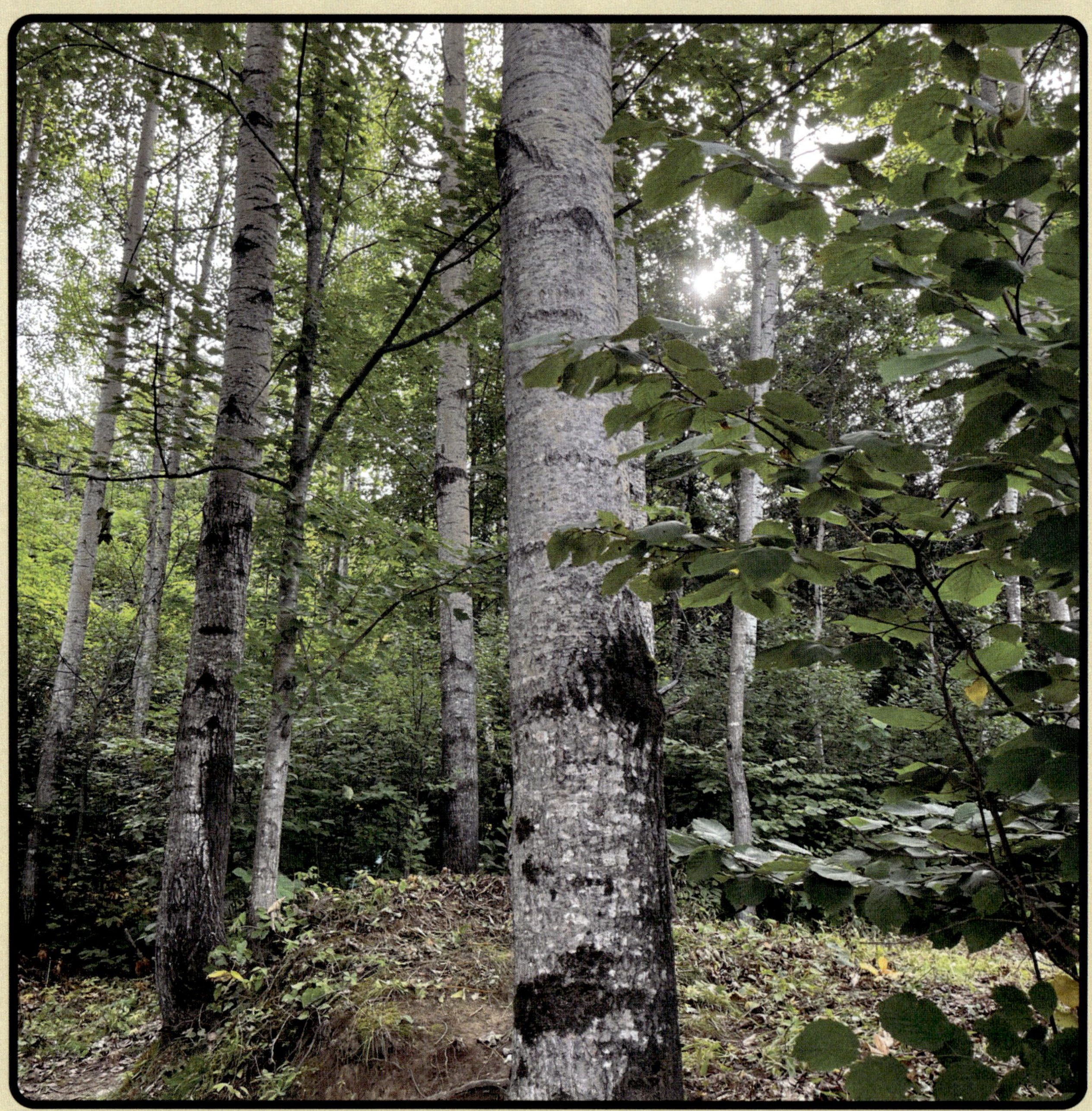

Bigtooth Aspen

Blooms: Ponatomuwi-kisuhs - Siqonomeqi-kisuhs (April - May)

Harvest time: Seeds are mature and ready to be harvested from Siqonomeqi-kisuhs - Niponi-kisuhs (May - June)

Medicinal uses: The bark of the tree can be used to treat rheumatism and fevers.

NOPISUNEKTUN

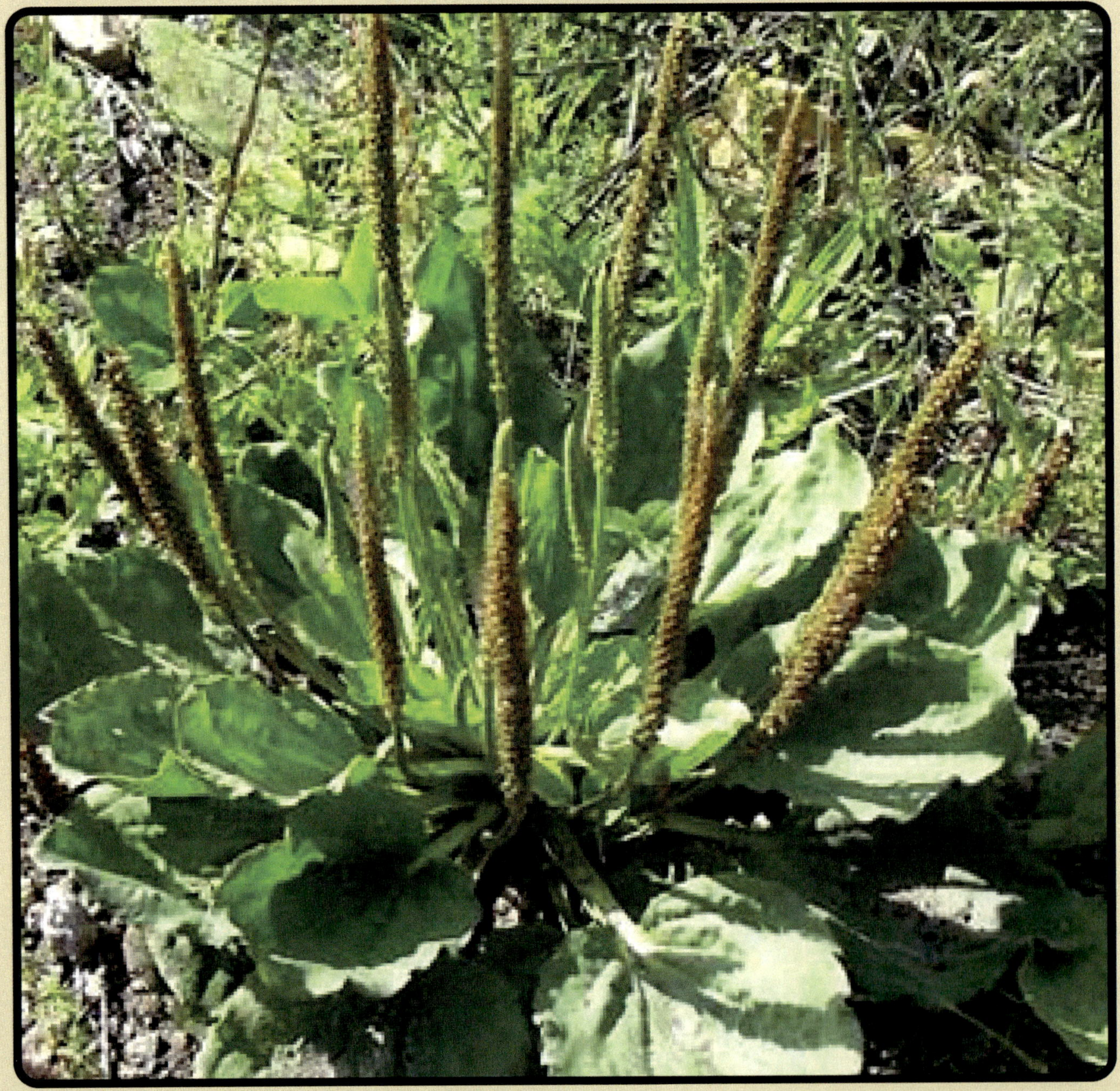

Plantain

Blooms: Most likely to bloom during siqoniw (spring) and/or niponiw (summer) because it's known to grow in poor rocky soil.

Harvest time: During the rainy seasons are the best time to harvest, ideally from Amilkewi-kisuhs - Ponatomuwi-kisuhs (October - April)

Medicinal use: It can be crushed or chewed and placed over the skin to heal bee stings, bug bites, acne, slivers, glass splinters, or rashes. Bandage the affected area afterwards and it will take 4-12 hours to heal. Plantain can be used as a balm for travel/emergency kits, or an infusion for skin or general wash. It can also be used for a smoothing remedy for hemorrhoids.

PUSPAHKOMIKEK

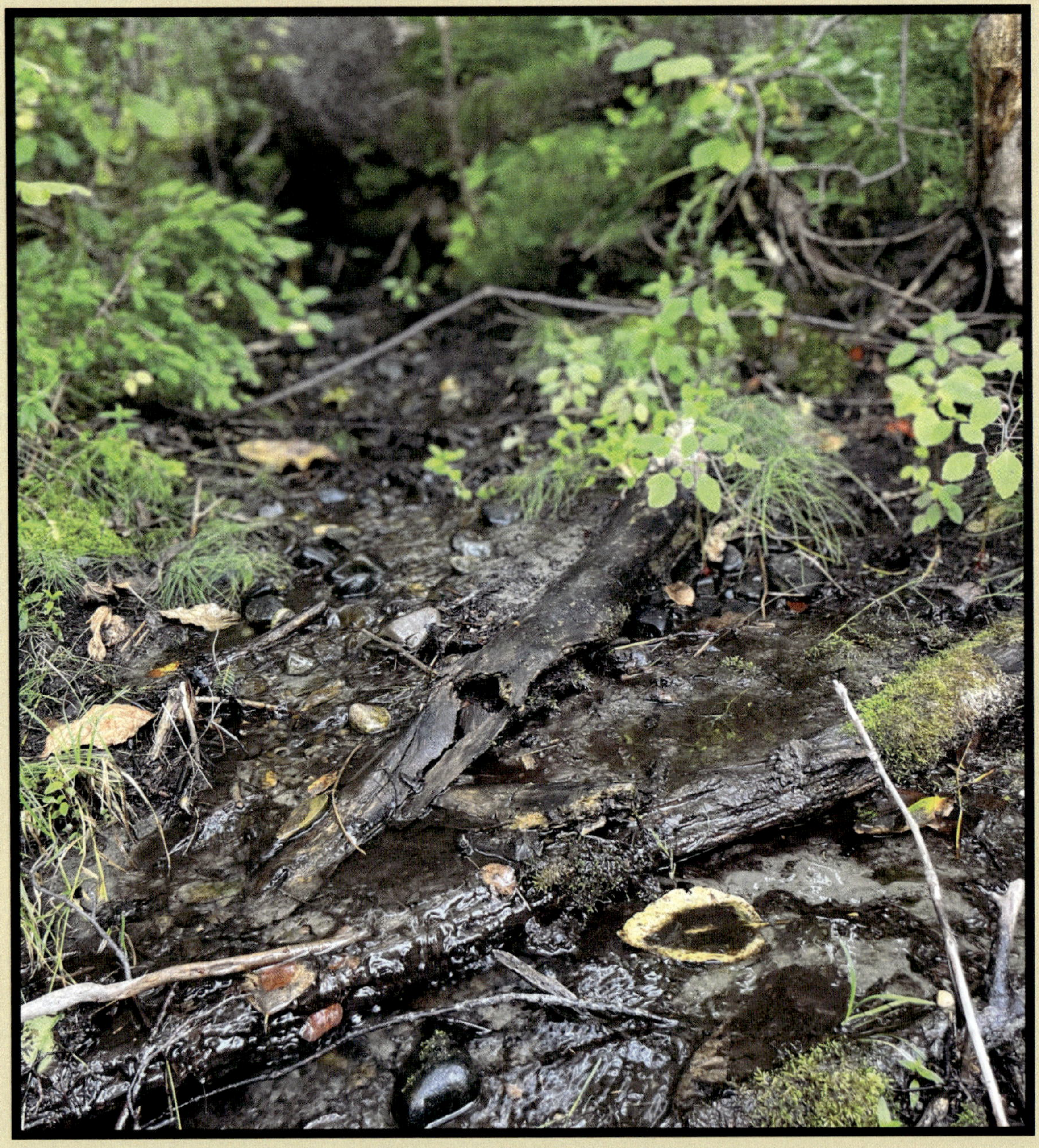

Marshlands

A marsh is a type of wetland that is dominated by grasses, animals, insects and other herbaceous plants such as cattails, water lilies, black spruce, red-winged black birds, muskrats, great blue heron, ducks, dragon flies, wood ticks, mosquitoes, and turtles.

They are highly productive and biologically diverse systems that enhance water quality, control erosion, maintain stream flows, isolate carbon, and provide a home to at least one third of all threatened and endangered species.

Made in the USA
Middletown, DE
29 January 2025

70508481R00022